# SEXUAL PENSÉES

# SEXUAL PENSÉES

## Bruce Jay Friedman

PLAYBOY PRESS
*New York, New York   Hanover, New Hampshire*

*"I used to like talking about sex . . .*
*to illustrate this fancy, I did, at one time,*
*consider a 'book of desire,' an anthology*
*of outlandish, melancholy and*
*droll stories about the subject."*

Narrator of *Blue, Blue Pictures of You,*
by Hanif Kureishi

For David Markson—whose work inspired this book—

*though he is by no means responsible for it.*

EDITED BY
*Michelle Urry*

DESIGNED BY
*Walter Bernard*

ILLUSTRATIONS BY
*André Barbe*

Copyright © 2006 by Playboy Enterprises International, Inc.
Illustrations copyright © 2006 by André Barbe

For information about permission to
reproduce selections from this book, write to
Playboy Press / Steerforth Press L.C., 25 Lebanon Street,
Hanover, New Hampshire 03755

LIBRARY OF CONGRESS CATALOGING-IN-PUBLICATION DATA
Friedman, Bruce Jay, 1930–
   Sexual pensées / Bruce Jay Friedman ; [illustrations by André Barbe]. — 1st ed.
      p.   cm.
   ISBN-10: 1-58642-120-4 (alk. paper); ISBN-13: 978-1-58642-120-5 (alk. paper)
   1. Sex — United States — Anecdotes.  2. Heterosexuality — United States.  I. Title.

HQ18.U5F74 2006
306.70973—dc22

                                    2006045585

FIRST EDITION

# Contents

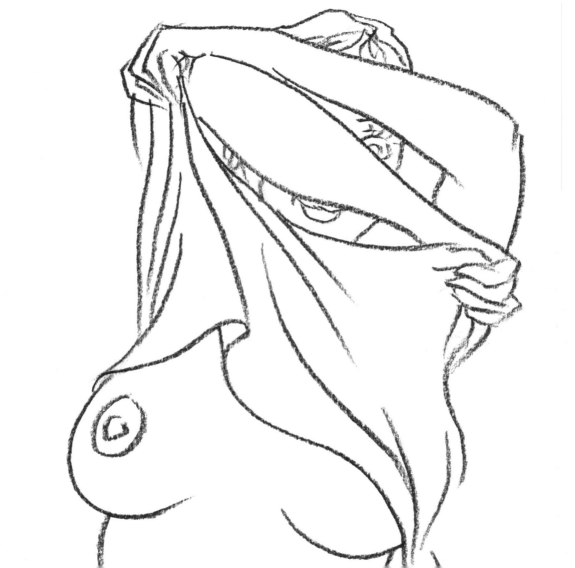

# Introduction

Not that he had been bombarded with offers to do so, but the author had on several occasions been asked why he had not written more directly about sex. He had covered a great deal of ground. His style had been described variously as being "supple," "sexual," even, on one occasion, as being "carnal." Yet he had never dealt with sex as a subject. However highly charged, wasn't it just another arena of behavior? Like politics? Or sports?

After quickly—and defensively—establishing that he enjoyed sex, he said that it did not particularly intrigue him as a topic, that it was all too personal—that others were more adept at it. Not for him the "iron staff," the "beckoning honeypot." What if he ended up on that awful list put out annually by the

British, "honoring" people who had done the worst writing about sex. What if he came in fourteenth? Would that be his legacy? And why, incidentally, was he so concerned about his legacy?

In the end (and that was another difficulty—the language began to do tricks) none of these explanations for his reluctance to take on the subject satisfied him. The country was awash with sex. It was impossible to begin the day and not run into a hailstorm of it. He had lived alone for a good twenty years in Manhattan. Why not heed the advice—not so much of Emerson and Rousseau—but of a studio executive who had once told him: "Nothing should be wasted"?

And so he decided to proceed—careful not to announce that he was going to "take a stab" at it, or, heaven forbid, "dip into" the subject.

Herewith,* a great many tales and observations that have been recalled, overheard, experienced, enhanced a bit here and there, and, for the most part, enjoyed. They represent moments in the lives of both women and men—and are drawn, more often than not, from years of living the merry—and often not-so-merry—single existence in Manhattan.

*Bruce Jay Friedman*
NEW YORK CITY

---

*The author's first—and inevitable—"herewith."

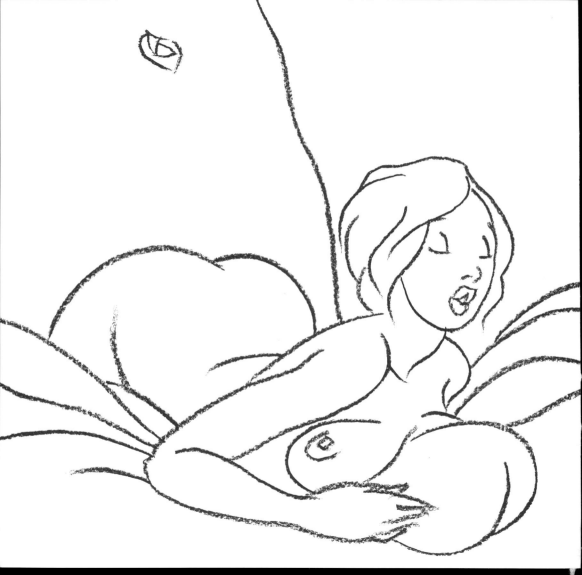

*Him*

**From time to time, he recalled a woman who waved—as if from a departing ship—before she went down on him.**

*The affair was proceeding at a congenial pace until she stretched out on his couch one night and said: "All right, spray my guts."*

Despondent after two nights of degradation in a brothel in Milan, he was consoled by another patron. "Do not despair," said the man. "This is the first step on the road back to God."
He did not believe this for a moment—but decided it was as good a place to start as any.

*He was seated beside a
celebrated actress at
a dinner party. Normally,
he would have reveled
in the experience. But
he'd heard it rumored that
at an early time in her
career, she had entertained
at a county fair, allowing
golf balls to be stroked
into her vagina.
No doubt he was being
overly fastidious, but
this spoiled the occasion
for him.*

There was no question that hair meant a great deal to him. He recalled a woman who enclosed him in what amounted to a tent of her long black tresses when they made love. Years later, she sent him a photograph of herself as a house-wife and mother, with short cropped hair. He barely recognized her and felt a certain sympathy for her husband.

**He found it off-putting when she referred to her vagina as a "knish."**

*When her memoir was published, naming the men she had slept with, he was relieved that he had not been mentioned. Then slowly, the disappointment set in.*

**He admired her clitoris, which was pink and perfectly shaped. "All right," she said. "But can we please not tell the world about it."**

A friend returned from South Beach in Miami and confessed he had been unable to catch the attention of any of the beautiful models who were at work there. But he had enjoyed great success with several women he described as being "one notch below."

From time to time, during their brief affair, she would transfer water slowly from her mouth into his—a procedure he found arousing. No doubt it was sexist of him, but years later, noting her swift rise as an executive in cable television, he wondered if it had anything to do with the water trick.

*His hopes of becoming a stand-up comic ended with his first performance—at college. A coed in the first row of the audience distracted him by crossing and uncrossing her legs; he forgot the point of his stories, fainted and had to be carried from the stage.*

**His first wife watched his every move with suspicion. His second wife never inquired as to his whereabouts or his activities. He remained faithful to his second wife.**

*A Tale of the Sixties*
Two pretty, waiflike creatures
approached him after a
concert at the Fillmore East
in Manhattan. They said they
had just arrived from San
Francisco and were without
money or a place to stay.
One said she had been the
lover of a noted rock
drummer—the other that
she always wore clean white
cotton underwear.
With no hesitation, he
decided to accommodate the
latter of the two.

**She had enormous breasts.
When he saw them he
was not only awestruck,
but mystified as to
how to deal with them.
"It's clear," she said,
turning away magisterially,
"that you've never
encountered a boobies girl."**

*Thoughout his life, he
had taken it for granted that
homely women would be
more receptive to his advances
than attractive ones.
More often than not, he was
mistaken.*

*He had met her only once and fell instantly and hopelessly in love with her. Deep in domestic crisis, he called her from a suburban skating rink while his daughters circled the ice. She agreed to meet him at the Plaza Hotel in Manhattan. When she failed to appear, he emptied the champagne—with some drama—into the sink. She kept the appointment fifteen years later, joining him in bed at the Plaza. Although he was no longer in love with her, he admired her for her sense of responsibility.*

**She was a beautiful woman who worked in a bank on the ground floor of a high-rise in which he lived. Several times a week they made love, during her lunch break. One day she showed up, distraught, and said that she had met someone she cared about.**

**"From now on," she said, "I will only be able to give you hand jobs."**

**He accepted her terms immediately.**

The size of his penis had never concerned him. It was bigger than his business partner's. That was enough.

*His first wife left him for another man. His second for a woman. He considered this to be progress.*

**It annoyed him that he had lost a woman he cared about to a herring czar.**

He was enamored of a strawberry-haired ballerina and pursued her relentlessly, to no avail. Later, he discovered that she had found him attractive—and would willingly have gone to bed with him—but was annoyed because he had never once come to see her dance.

*Only once had he been able to ejaculate repeatedly over the course of an evening.*

*He'd met the woman at a crowded bistro. She stumbled— he ran to assist her. They returned to his flat and made love, again and again, throughout the night. No sooner had he come than he would be erect again.*

*How was this possible?*

*Was it her eyes, which were a striking color of blue? Her lean model's body?*

*Or his awareness that she was scheduled to leave for Italy in the morning? And that it was unlikely he would ever see her again?*

*For all of his bravado, he refused to allow a pretty, young, female physician to examine his prostate.*

**He stopped watching porno films when he realized they had created an expectation that every woman he met would, within minutes, fall to her knees and begin cheerfully to suck his penis.**

A dark moment in his life came about when he was no longer sleeping with his wife and she was preparing to leave him. It was not helpful when their mutual friend, who was painfully beautiful, turned to him at a dinner party and complained that she was bored with *her* marriage.

"All we do is fuck," she said. "Surely there's more to life than that."

*When his psychiatrist died,*
*he decided to continue his*
*treatment with a woman, his*
*freewheeling style having never*
*been exposed to a female*
*point of view. During his first*
*session, he mentioned*
*that he made occasional visits*
*to a prostitute.*
*"Oh, my God," the therapist*
*said with revulsion.*
*"You've got to stop doing*
*that immediately."*

**Overheard at a hotel bar in Miami Beach: "I can understand him sleeping with my wife— but my *mother*?"**

*Remarks from Women that Lingered:*

- Call me if you're ever in the mood for an affair.

- It appears I'm just another chapter in your book.

- I'm up for a fuck if you are.

- Oh, my God, you're worshiping my ass.

- I don't understand . . . my last lover had no trouble getting it in.

- Relax. I'll sleep with you. But let's have dinner first.

> *She excused herself to take a call from her lover,*
> *a utility infielder for a major league baseball*
> *team. Had the man been in the starting lineup,*
> *he might, respectfully, have gotten to his*
> *feet and lit a cigarette. As it was, he continued,*
> *snobbishly, to lick her vagina.*

**He admired the courage of a woman
who had placed an ad in the personals,
saying that she was intelligent
and accomplished, "though not a beauty."
But he did not respond to the ad.**


A letter to the editor of *Cosmopolitan*:

Dear *Cosmo,*

      Your article in the November issue ("Big Butt Be Gone")
fails to take into account a considerable group of us out here
who admire, and even *prefer,* a big butt now and then. Shapely,
of course. We are not talking "lard-ass" here. But substantial?
Absolutely.

                    Sincerely,
                    BJF
                    Southampton, NY

He insisted—to his friends—that there were transvestites in Miami
who were more beautiful—and feminine—than any woman.
"They can fool you totally," he said.
But in his one experience, he had not been fooled.

*As he chatted casually with a grande
dame—in a literary salon—the woman
suddenly hoisted her legs above
her head and locked her ankles behind
her neck. The maneuver, as far as
he could tell, was unrelated to any topic
under discussion.*
*Though, happily, she was wearing
slacks at the time, he could not erase
the tableau from his memory.*

**He found it amusing
when she shaved her
pubic hair, but
it did not prolong their
affair significantly.**

*Late one night, an attractive woman with whom he'd*
*had a brief affair knocked on his apartment door,*
*rousing him from a deep sleep. Clearly distressed (she'd*
*been quarreling with her current lover), she asked*
*if he would perform oral sex on her. Though he was*
*only half-awake, he accommodated her nonetheless.*
*But when she left the apartment, he began, for the*
*first time, to question his lifestyle.*

**A friend complained that although he**
**asked an escort service to send only blue-eyed**
**blondes to his apartment, they repeatedly**
**ignored his instructions. Instead, they**
**dispatched a series of tall black transvestites.**
**When asked if he sent them back,**
**he refused to comment.**

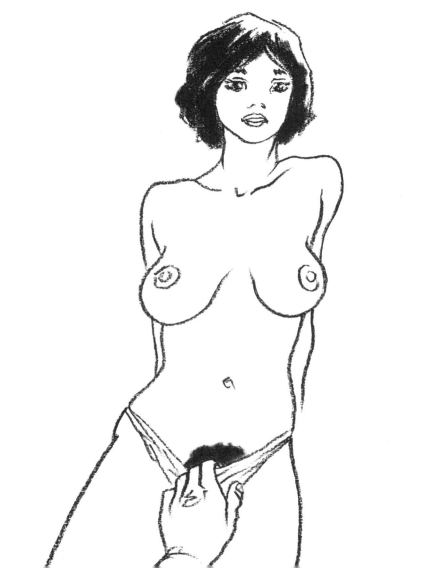

*Her*

*She was reading an
English mystery novel beside
the hotel pool when a
young man approached her.
"My friend would like
to know," he said, pointing
to a second man on the
terrace, "if you're married,
engaged or tied up with
anyone at the moment."
"None of the above," she
said. "Tell him to come over
and stick it in."*

At an international monetary
conference, she went to
bed with an economist from the
Republic of Georgia. Though it
was absurd of her to think this
way, she was surprised that
men from that part of the world
made love in much the same
manner as their American
counterparts. (That they enjoyed
cunnilingus, for example.)
She shared her experience with
a gay colleague.
"Why, darling," he said,
"the Republic of Georgia is the
home of cunnilingus."

**Her only complaint about her lover was that he never said anything filthy to her in bed. But it was a major complaint.**

*She was seated beside a socialite who was said to be a descendant of the early settlers at Plymouth Rock. "What do you do in life?" he asked. As a lark, she replied: "I'm a retired porno star." He turned away frostily and said no more to her throughout the dinner. But as she got up from the table, he asked if she was involved with anyone at the moment.*

She had a recurring fantasy of being taken suddenly and roughly (though willingly) in the style of the bodice-ripping novels she enjoyed. But when the scenario became a reality, she found the results disappointing. The man, an insurance agent, was attractive enough, but was only half-erect throughout. And before he left her flat, he attempted to sell her an endowment policy.

*She'd had a brief affair with*
*a professor. Each night she would*
*arrive at his flat, fully dressed*
*for dinner. After a civilized interval,*
*she would cross the room in*
*silence, lift her skirt, straddle him—*
*and he would enter her.*
*Only in this manner did they*
*make love.*
*But it was enough.*

**Though she knew better—and there was evidence to the contrary—she felt that she could seduce the occasional gay man who attracted her.**

And though it was violative of current thought,
she preferred a large penis to a small one.

Though she had never experienced anal sex, she was curious about it. So one morning, when he suggested they try it, she did not discourage him. No sooner had he entered her than the phone rang. He pulled away to answer it.

"I can't believe this," she said indignantly. "The first time I have anal sex and you're taking *calls*?"

**She admitted candidly to an interviewer on Italian televison that she had stopped writing novels for a decade because of a total preoccupation with sex and drugs. Actually, it was two decades.**

A Tale of the Seventies
*She was one of the first applicants for a job as a waitress in a new Manhattan restaurant. In order to be hired, she was told, she would have to give oral sex to the owner. She declined—and was disturbed by the experience. Even more so when she noted how quickly the restaurant had become fully staffed.*

*She was scheduled to meet a boy she had been dating—*
*and felt uneasy about doing so since she had fallen in love*
*with another student. When she arrived at the boy's*
*dorm he introduced her to his parents, who were*
*visiting from out of state. She found them pinched and*
*uncommunicative, almost blatantly rude.*
*Later, the boy said his parents wanted him to stop seeing*
*her—having learned that she was Jewish. Offering*
*no rebuttal, she said she understood. She wished him well*
*and drove off.*
*Never had she dreamed that anti-Semitism could have its*
*positive aspects.*

**She was distracted—and did poorly—in a job interview, having become convinced that she had seen the interviewer perform in a porno movie.**

*To amuse her lover, and because she felt he was about to leave her, she arranged for her roommate to join them in bed.*
*"But remember," she warned him, "you only come in your girlfriend."*

She wondered about the *coup de foudre*—a powerful phenomenon in which one meets an individual and falls instantly and hopelessly in love. Though it was said to occur once in a lifetime, she felt it had happened to her at least fifty times.

She met him at a museum and quickly discovered that they shared the same surname. His features and his coloring, too, were similar to hers. Later, when she touched his skin, it was as if she was touching her own. Making love to him was like making love to herself. But if this was interesting, that was *all* that was interesting. He became abusive, refused to leave her apartment and had to be removed by the building superintendent.

*It was her feeling that men from the South were more ebullient and demonstrative about sex.*
*She recalled a man from Mississippi crying out:"Great God in heaven and hallelujah, you are removing your panties."*

**Though she admired her lover's penis, it reminded her—in its erect state— of a puppet.**

*She had been determined to lose her virginity before she turned twenty-one and was pleased to have accomplished her goal. Save for the fact that her lover turned up in flowered bikini underwear, the experience was uneventful.*

A celebrated hairstylist disapproved of her recent behavior. "You've been acting like a slut," he said. She stormed out of his salon. But the stylist had great skills. Her vanity was unlimited. She soon scheduled another appointment.

**A young man she slept with kept withdrawing— during intercourse— to thank her for the "gift" she was bestowing upon him. This brought down the encounter considerably.**

She would have found it tacky
if a stranger, no matter how
attractive, had asked her
the color of her panties.
Such was not the case with
her roommate, who found such
inquiries charming.

**She decided—in the Nineties—to eliminate from her life anyone who said "Ciao" upon parting.**

*She could not derive pleasure from the sex scenes in a novel (no matter how skillfully rendered) if the author's dust jacket photograph did not appeal to her.*

*Though legally of age, he was a little watch fob of a man.*
*A powerful woman, she was able to twirl his naked body about*
*while he chuckled back at her. She had never made love*
*to one of her students before, but she felt, in this one case, she*
*would be forgiven.*

They made love at length and gymnastically.
They used several motorized items. At her
request, he tied her to a bed with scarves and
spanked her with a salmon that had been
reserved for their dinner.
Still, she left in a pique, saying: "Nothing
kinky ever happens to me."

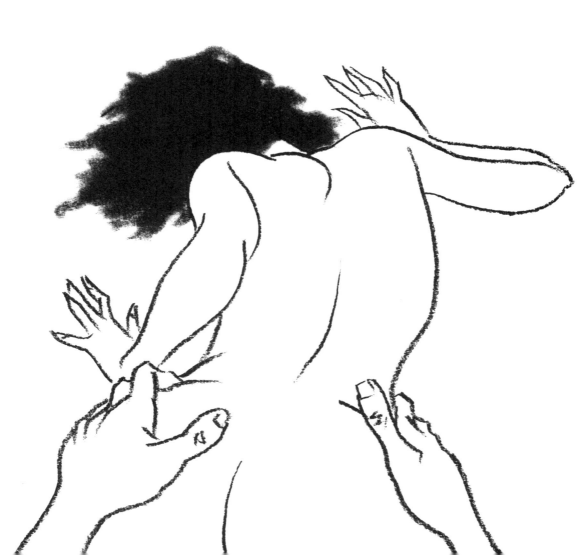

*Them*

She was a model who did most of her work in Italy. They had a brief affair. One day, as they were making love in a Southampton cottage they'd rented for the weekend, she suddenly broke away, gathered her things and left. He confronted her at a party several years later and asked her how she could do something so unsportsmanlike. "I know, I know," she said. "It was rude of me. But I was in the middle of a career change. And not to worry. I owe you half a fuck."

*She was a big, rawboned, hearty woman from the South. They spent exactly one big, rawboned and hearty night in bed. He remembered her primarily for some advice she had given him: "Before you go out on a date, put a drop of cologne on your crotch area. Women find this irresistible." From time to time, he followed this instruction, with only mixed results. Perhaps, he concluded, it was more effective with women from the South.*

The model he dated took pride in being well-read, a rarity, she
claimed, in her profession. Nonetheless, he began to take
notice of other models who worked for the agency.
"You wouldn't like them," she said. "They're all stupid. They
do nothing but lie around and have their legs waxed."
It was one of the great mistakes of his life that he believed her.

**"We've been eyeing each other all night," she said,
from a booth adjacent to his at a crowded
restaurant. "So we might as well get acquainted."
As it happened, he had not noticed her before; she
was a plain, somewhat homely-looking woman.
But the audacity of her invitation was appealing.
At the end of the evening, he left with her.**

Though she was more than obliging in this area, his mistress claimed that women did not truly enjoy giving oral sex—and did it only as an accommodation to their lovers. To support her position, she said she had canvassed her girlfriends on the subject. Assuming this was true, he found it remarkable how often he had been fooled.

**His new mistress confided that she had slept with more than two hundred men. He understood the appeal of sexually experienced women, but in this case, he felt the numbers were excessive.**

*She had delicate features and short, streaky, blonde hair. She was a most unlikely drug dealer. "Gamine" is the word that suited her. After a delivery to his apartment, they began to make love. The form it took is that they would lie still, for long periods of time, his mouth on her vagina, hers enclosing his penis. Later, he discovered that she lived with an 80-year-old black man who was blind. He wondered if she and the black man made love in the same manner. And was it the black man who had taught her that style?*

**Women popping freely into (occupied) men's rooms, men doing the reverse. It was a scenario that seemed emblematic of the Seventies.**

After they had spent the night in her apartment—making love— they spoke about buying a house— and spending their lives together. They would be inseparable. They were quiet for a moment. She asked then if she could hold his supply of cocaine until their next meeting. He refused, feeling that such an arrangement represented too great a commitment.

*During a routine trip to the supermarket, he decided—on an impulse—to stop off and see a former girlfriend who lived nearby. They made love—all of which took no more than twenty minutes. When he returned to his apartment, the picture of what he felt was innocence, his mistress stopped him at the door. "Do that again," she said, "and I'll kill you."*

*With no apparent source of income, she lived in a magnificent townhouse in Greenwich Village. The walls were covered with photographs of her in the nude. One night, she confided in him that she was being sponsored by a wealthy older man. "All that he requires is that I join him on his yacht— once a year—and massage his prostate on the high seas." He felt this was a reasonable arrangement, but would have preferred that she had not told him the story.*

The poet had brought his German girlfriend along to the symposium and seemed to be offering her around to his colleagues. The woman, in turn, helped the scenario along by indicating that she was available. "I take my panties off to you, sir," was a typical remark of hers. There was a feeling that if anyone had accepted the offer, the poet would have torn out his throat.

*He became obsessed by the black and white photograph of a nude woman in a magazine—and went to great lengths to track her down to a house in suburban New Jersey. He offered to pay her a substantial sum of money to re-create the pose for him in her living room. She was suspicious at first and concerned that her husband might soon arrive. But she was impressed by all the trouble the stranger had taken to locate her. She agreed, finally, to strip off her nightgown and to strike the coveted pose for him—but only after negotiating a higher fee.*

**After chatting casually with a young woman he'd met at a bar, he asked if she would like to have dinner with him one night. "It depends," she said, "on what you mean by dinner."**

In the early stages of their affair, she would fall to her knees and suck his penis—before allowing him to venture out into the night. He was aware of being "controlled," but could not bring himself to ask that she discontinue the practice.

*He presented his theory to a woman he had just*
*met in a cocktail lounge.*
*"Sex is simply one more arena of behavior.*
*What happens between a man and a woman in*
*bed proceeds naturally from what's come before.*
*There are no surprises."*
*The woman looked at him in astonishment.*
*Everything that had ever happened to her*
*in bed had come as a surprise.*

**A girl named Maureen stood on the top rung of**
**some climbing bars. He got his first glimpse of**
**panties, white and torn. And he guessed correctly**
**that he was fated to marry an Irish girl.**

An attractive divorcée he had met at a party invited him
back to her handsomely decorated apartment on
Sutton Place. Upon arriving, she went immediately to her
kitchen and began to boil a substance he later learned
was crack cocaine.
She sifted, ground and shaped the resulting material,
then stuffed it into a pipe. Anticipating a night of unbridled
sex, he joined her in taking a few puffs and was thrown
off stride when she said: "Hold me. All I want is to be held."
Unable to hide his disappointment, he reminded her
that it had taken a good part of an hour to prepare the
concoction they were smoking. "We didn't have to go to all
that trouble. I would have held you without the drug."
"All right then," she said resignedly. "You can rub my feet."

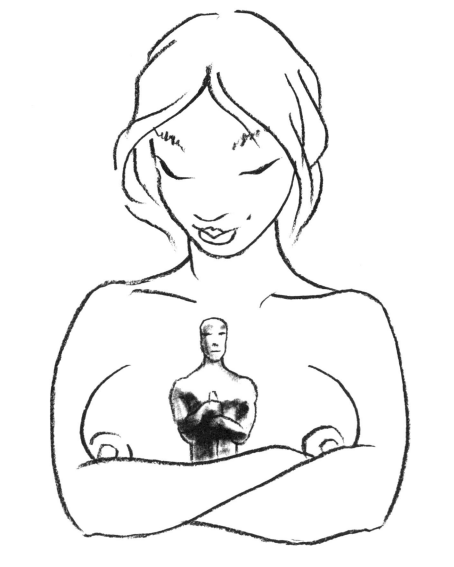

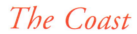

*The Coast*

*After they had known each other for a year, she began silently—during sexual intercourse—to compose Academy Awards acceptance speeches. She took this as a sign that their affair was losing its intensity.*

**The starlet arrived at a Hollywood party and was greeted at the door by the host, who asked her to suck his cock. "I left," she told friends, "since I was not at his level of partying."**

A film producer who had been married and divorced four times made an announcement to his lunch companions. "I have finally met the woman of my dreams. She is a retired Israeli tank commander who sells real estate in Beverly Hills." Within weeks, the two were circling each other with knives. His friends were not surprised.

*She decided not to hire a Hollywood agent whose proposal had been as follows: "Let me represent you and I'll spread your name across this town like manure."*

**An agent told her that "the people around Steven Spielberg" were interested in her as an actress. "But what about Spielberg himself?" she asked. "We're researching that," said the agent.**

Her friends became concerned when the starlet, who was generally jolly and upbeat, appeared to be low in spirits. She explained that while she was en route to the Academy Awards ceremony in a limousine, her date, an Albanian, had come on her neck.

The producer stood up at a script conference, excused himself to the assembled writers, undressed and joined a young woman in his guest room for a period of twenty minutes.
When he returned, wearing a robe, he was gasping, ashen-faced and seemed to be near death. "I only do this," he told the writers, "because I know you fellows expect it of me."

*In a show of self-assertion, the starlet told her friends she no longer slept with an actor she had been dating—because of his abusive behavior toward her. "Of course I still give him head," she said. "After all, he* is *a movie star."*

**"I'm a pure screenwriter," said her dinner companion at a Hollywood party. "You just play at it. That's the difference between you and I."**

During the Cannes Film Festival, the producer rented an entire bordello for his exclusive use—and had the women service him, one by one, throughout the night. Later, he accepted his therapist's explanation that his behavior was neurotic and had nothing to do with sex—but he refused to regret the experience.

**The starlet described what she did in Hollywood swimming pools as "light screwing."**

*At Morton's restaurant in Los Angeles, she had lunch with a director whose recent film had failed at the box office. After drinks, he sat back expansively and formed a circle with his arms, as if to describe a tree trunk.*
*"I feel," he said, "as if my cock is this big."*
*She wondered how big his cock would have felt if his film had been successful.*

**The starlet told her agent she refused to do full-frontal nudity. "However," she added, "my tush is negotiable."**

She had written a screenplay about a woman whose husband runs off with a beautiful young black woman. Soon afterward, her husband ran off with a beautiful young black woman.
This caused her—from then on—to consider her choice of subject more carefully.

**As his dying wish, an eighty-seven year-old film producer asked to be taken on a tour of Manhattan's sex clubs.**

*A college roommate, who was visiting from New York, arrived back at her friend's Beverly Hills apartment in a distraught state. She had made a date with a film star. When she arrived at his hotel suite, he asked her if she would like to "taste his ass" before they went out to dinner.*
*"I don't know why you're upset," she told her college roommate. "It sounds like a fairly representative Hollywood first date to me."*

After the producer's third use of the word *pullulate* (i.e., "various projects pullulated before my eyes") she decided she could never accept him as a lover. But she had a strong sense that his liberal use of the word had contributed to his prominence in Hollywood.

**The producer was famed—not so much for the movies he had made, but for his reputation of making love to aging screen stars while he sat beside them and watched their early films on television.**

She extricated herself from a tight situation (a producer had cornered her in his Beverly Hills hotel suite) by warning him that she had been trained by the Mossad. "My 'kill time,'" she said, "has been certified at eight seconds." Upon hearing this, he backed off and asked if she would like to have some dinner.

*He attended a weekly poker game in Santa Monica during which the late-night conversation would veer off now and then to the subject of blow jobs. Great blow jobs. Memorable ones. The perfect blow job. He was not taken seriously—and was indeed hooted down—when he said with all sincerity that he had personally never experienced a bad one.*

**To impress her, the producer said that he had slept with hundreds of women. "McDonald's," she said with a shrug, "sells lots of hamburgers."**

The producer had been that rarity in Hollywood—a family man, a loving husband, the devoted father of four children. Yet one night he succumbed to temptation and arranged to meet an actress in a suite at the Beverly Hills Hotel. Learning of the planned tryst, his wife burst in upon the fully clothed couple, demanded and won a divorce—and left the producer a broken man at sixty.

They were leaving her small apartment in Manhattan when he suddenly became crazed by the look of her. For the first time in their affair, he tore off her clothing and penetrated her anally. Thinking he had violated her, he was appalled by his behavior. Unperturbed, she had pulled up her blue jeans and said: "Thanks. I needed that."

At that moment, he predicted—correctly as it turned out—that she would become a major force in Hollywood.

**He lost respect for his psychiatrist when she abandonned her patients—some of them suicidal—to become an executive at Warner Brothers.**

*In Malibu one summer, he thought he had found the ultimate starlet: yellow hair, green eyes, freckles, all of it. But when she asked him to post bond for her teenage brothers who were under indictment for armed robbery, he decided to end their brief affair.*

*At his weekly poker game, a screenwriter told with pride of having written a successful role for a celebrated Italian actress. She expressed her gratitude by cooking a bowl of spaghetti for him. All in attendance agreed it would have been a better story if she had taken him to bed.*

A woman accepted his invitation to spend two weeks with him at the Chateau Marmont in California. The time spent was blissful. But upon their return to Manhattan, she learned that her dog had died during her absence—and held him responsible.

**Holding court in a Santa Monica restaurant, a Hollywood mogul insisted for years that women who wanted to meet him must first place a hand on his ancient penis.**

*"I can show you London,"*
*said the producer. "Paris, Rome,*
*places you've never been."*
*"But I was born in Paris," said*
*the young woman. "I grew up in*
*Italy and worked in London*
*for three years."*
*"Yes," said the producer, undeterred.*
*"But did you ever really* see *them?"*

**"Pretend you are doing it for the first time." These were the words she heard from a film star with whom she was spending the night in bed. It was not until the next morning that she realized he was giving her an acting tip.**

On a busy street in Manhattan, he noticed a film star he knew slightly, soliciting women as they left a popular department store. This surprised him. The man was known to have had affairs with some of the most beautiful women in the world—and presumably could have had his pick of others.

"The way I look at it," the star explained, "if I can score one out of eight, I'm ahead of the game."

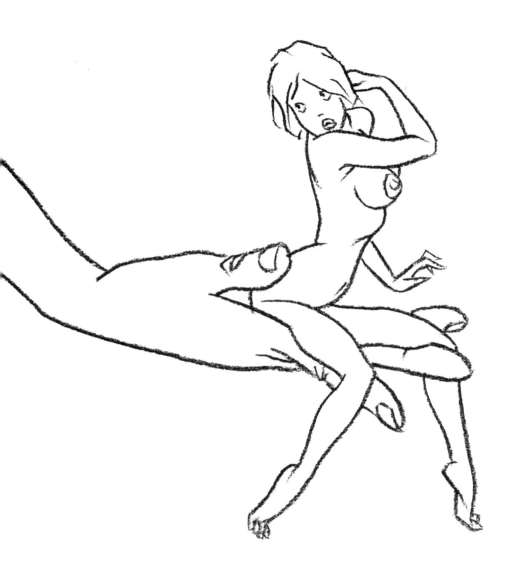

*Icons*

*At a dinner party, he was seated beside an elderly woman who had enjoyed a distinguished career in the State Department. After several drinks, he told her of his lifelong infatuation with women of every age, shape and variety.*
*"You make a mistake," she said languorously, "when you underestimate pussy power."*

**In an interview with the *New York Times*, the actress Natasha Richardson said she realized, while performing in a Broadway musical, that a man in the front row had a clear view up her dress—somehow implying that the man was at fault.**

In a letter to someone named "James," Ernest Hemingway's third wife, Martha Gellhorn, described a mutual acquaintance: "He is whipped cream fun to be with." The use of this phrase, the reader felt, was grounds for divorce.

*Tennessee Williams complimented the actress on her perfect skin. "Yes," she said, seizing an opportunity to quote from one of his works, "but I'm a prisoner within it."*

**She met Calvin Klein at a cocktail party and said she was a great fan of his underwear.**

After they had slept together, the woman said:
"Now that we have that out of the way, we can commence to be friends."
He was charmed by the remark and disappointed when he learned that she had been paraphrasing the novelist Mary McCarthy.

Choose Your Own Philosophy Department:
- *Lead a circumspect life and be wild in your imagination.* —FLAUBERT
- *It is dangerous to lead a safe life.* —NIETZSCHE

*Though dreams—particularly those of others—were less than fascinating to her, she did have a recurring one she found intriguing. In the dream, she is carrying former Secretary of State Madeleine Albright on her back, through a rockslide in the Grand Canyon.*

*"Hang on, Madame Secretary," she says, as boulders crash all about them. "I'll get you through."*

*"Thank you," Albright replies. "You are a fine American."*

**During the Clinton Administration sex scandal, he asked the pretty young secretary in an adjoining office what she thought of the president's predicament. Correctly guessing his motivation, she said: "You're only asking so you can hear me say the words *blow job*."**

When his wife began to have affairs, he sought out—for no other reason than that— lovers of his own.

A wise friend counseled him: "Do not attempt to compete with a woman on that level. You will always lose."

She had some difficulty with the actor Paul Newman's response to an interviewer's question about marital infidelity. "Why eat hamburger when you've got steak at home?" Undeniably, the sentiment was commendable. But wasn't it unfair to those who prefer hamburger?

**She was familiar with the observation of philosophers: consummation of the sex act is not half so pleasurable as the lustful anticipation of it. But her experience did not bear this out.**

**A distinguished-looking gentleman he met at a café in Rome claimed that as an Italian prisoner of war (captured by Americans in World War II) he had been forced to give oral sex to the Andrews Sisters.**

*In a televised debate having to do with human sexuality, she was alarmed to find herself quoting not only Friedrich Nietzsche, but also the actress Sharon Stone.*

In the course of an interview with the late—and quite brilliant—novelist Terry Southern, a journalist gave his opinion that, in terms of satisfying a woman, there was no substitute for the penis.

Whereupon Southern thrust a fist in front of the interviewer's nose and said: "What about *this*?"

**Why was it necessary for him to learn—in the press—that Barbra Streisand and James Brolin slept in the spoon position?**

*Once he had discovered that Freud sought out the company of prostitutes, he felt better about his own tendencies in that direction. The same, of course, was true of cocaine.*

*Mario Puzo was told of a colleague who had died suddenly.*
*For years he had given up his vices—and led a healthy life.*
*Said the novelist: "It was that life without vice that killed him.*
*"And I don't understand why vice has such a bad reputation,"*
*Puzo continued. "My vices are all that I've ever enjoyed."*

She had great fondness for the words of General Auguste-Alexandre Ducrot, who had been rushed to Sedan (during the Franco-Prussian War of 1870) to review the hopeless battlefield situation of the surrounded French army.

After one look at the map he is reported to have said:

*"Nous somme dans le pot de chambre . . . et nous y serons emmerdes."*

("We are in the toilet . . . and they are going to shit on us.")

*"When two people part, it is the one who is not in love who makes the tender speeches."*

—MARCEL PROUST

Though he admired Proust, he could not recall his wife making tender speeches when she left him.

**Nothing infuriated Mario Puzo more than people who sought counseling for sex addiction. "They should get down on their knees and thank god they have such an affliction."**

Puzo sympathized with a friend who had enjoyed great success with women but was now old and infirm. The friend assured him that age has its compensations.
"For the first time in my life, I can be with a beautiful woman and be confident that she has no power over me."

"Never sleep with a woman who has more troubles than you do." —NELSON ALGREN

*It occurred to her that had she applied this dictum to the men in her life, she would have remained a virgin.*

*Arriving at a college campus to participate in a symposium, the editor of a scholarly journal looked about at all the pretty coeds.*
*"This is one more town,"*
*he said despairingly, "in which I am not going to get laid."*

**Picasso's *Guernica* was awesome—but no more so to him than the sight of a woman pushing a lock of her hair behind her ear, as preparation for (delivering) oral sex.**

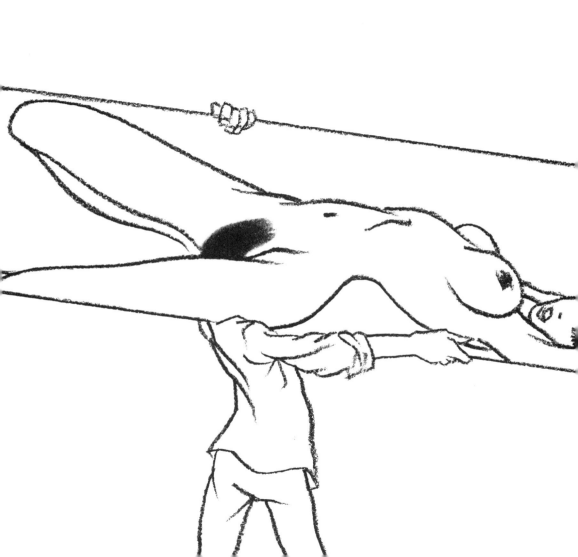

*Him (2)*

He continued to live with a woman who had become fat—
for fear that if he left, she would immediately become
thin again. But his concern was not justified. Eventually, he
did leave her—and learned from friends that she had
had the good grace to have remained fat.

**He insisted on
being compared
to her other lovers.
After some
consideration, she
said he was the
most "thorough,"
which was not the
description he
preferred.**

*A woman he had known took pride
in being able to click off virtually
motorized contractions with her
vagina during intercourse. He found
this amusing, but it did not alter
his life significantly. Nor did it
prolong their affair.*

*Does Oral Sex Qualify as a Sexual Act?*
At the time of the White House sex scandal, he raised this question to a friend at a bar in the West Village. And was amazed by the enthusiasm with which women on all sides joined the discussion— and how passionately they pursued the subject, until all hours of the night.

*Why was it that there was only one woman with whom he'd enjoyed phone sex? Was it because she was a good listener? And responded with enthusiasm? And lived in an adjacent building? And that he could induce her from time to time (after much begging and pleading) to come to his apartment and sleep with him? Or was it because she was a high-powered agent for hockey stars?*

**He was no stranger to the naked female form. But his first sight of a topless sunbather—from his hotel room window in St. Tropez— was erotic to the point of taking away his sanity.**

Though he was heterosexual ("openly heterosexual" is the phrase
he used) he was invited to the opening of a gay nightclub.
And thought, as a lark, that he would try to establish his value,
so to speak, in the marketplace.
But he took offense when he was asked to dance by a short Lebanese
man who had garlic on his breath and wore a bad suit.

*His mistress, upon discovering that he had been*
*having an affair with a German woman:*
*Do you love her?*
*No.*
*Yet you sleep with her.*
*Yes.*
*Why?*
*To punish her.*
*Why not punish me?*
*You're not a German.*

**He was puzzled by
his interest in a drab and
somewhat innocuous-
looking woman in his
office—and decided that
she was a great deal
prettier than she let on.**

**He agreed to parade in front of his mistress in the nude, thinking it only sporting—since he had often made the same request of her. But he was unprepared for her suggestion that he lose a few pounds.**

He had not taught for some time. When he did, the weeklong experience left him drained and exhausted. After he completed his function, he visited a topless bar in Montreal and became intrigued by a slender young dancer. He offered to pay her to go back to his hotel and sleep with him. She resisted—and did not agree until he offered her his entire stipend for the week's work. When he realized what he had done, he felt ridiculous. But when he awakened the next morning, he was refreshed and invigorated.

*As a young bachelor in New York, he was treated by a dental hygienist who also provided him with a full social agenda—arranging dates for him with her many attractive girlfriends. But it was the hygienist herself, with her fresh smile and magical hands, who interested him—and she was unavailable.*

During a business trip to Stockholm, he called his
mistress and said that after a week of being surrounded by
blondes, he began to long for a dark-haired woman.
His mistress had dark hair.
And from time to time he found it necessary to lie to her.

It troubled him that on a night candlelight vigils were being held in support of the besieged novelist Salman Rushdie, he was seated at a bar in Jacksonville, Florida, trying to talk a cocktail waitress into going to bed with him.

*A poet himself, it infuriated him that he had lost a woman to a rival who merely read aloud to her the poetry of others. (Later, when he regained some perspective, he conceded that the poetry his rival had selected was of the highest order— much more accomplished than any- thing he himself had written.)*

**He was dogged in his pursuit of women—and frustrated that he could not bring the same intensity to his tennis game.**

When he told the story, he said that it was a single remark she'd made that caused him to take notice of her—and led to their affair. He had been holding forth at a party, saying there were no longer any foods you could trust—except perhaps lima beans. "Haven't you heard about lima beans?" she asked.
But in telling the story, he said nothing about her yellow hair and blue eyes.

*A friend asked if he would look up a woman in London who might be in need of company. He agreed to do so. When he arrived at her flat, she flew at him and tore at his clothing in the manner of love-starved women in novels that were set in the tropics. Months later his friend called and said that, although he was generally a decent man, his London behavior proved him a swine when it came to women.*

Unaccountably, he continued to think back to an encounter he'd had— as a young man—with a pretty young prostitute in Stockholm. Sheepishly, he had asked what was expected of him. "We are here," she'd said, somewhat professorially, "for the purpose of sexual intercourse."

*He was not entirely sure of what a "forensic accountant" did. But when he learned that his wife had hired one, he agreed immediately to see a counselor and try to repair the marriage.*

**A Wall Street trader with whom he had spent the night unsettled him by sitting up suddenly in bed and announcing— fiercely—"I *must* have this four times a week."**

He was about to place an ad in the personals, saying he wanted to meet a young woman who was witty and charming and had "mischief" in her eyes—when he realized that he lived with just such a woman.

**With regard to the Winter Olympics, was he alone in concentrating not so much on the grace and beauty of the women skaters, but on their dazzling white panties?**

*His psychiatrist had an unusual proposal. He had attended a convention and met a beautiful young sex researcher who was visiting from Sweden.*
*"She's staying at a hotel in Manhattan and could use some company. Why don't you call her?"*
*When he declined, saying that he was dating several women at the time, the psychiatrist lost his composure and threw a paperweight at him.*

Prior to attending a symposium in Bogotá, he joined a group of academics who decided to visit a local bordello. No sooner had they entered the premises than the most prominent of them—a leading literary deconstructionist—sat on the lap of a fat prostitute, thrust his tongue down her throat and then disappeared with the woman—never to be seen again for the duration of the conference.

**When a friend accused him of having an affair with the man's wife, he was vigorous in his denial. To his way of thinking, a one-night stand did not constitute an affair.**

*An office worker he admired paid absolutely no attention to him. Yet when he turned up at a company function with his wife, she managed to get him aside and to brush her hand lightly against his crotch.*

*As he prepared to leave a party in Greenwich Village, he noticed that his raincoat was missing. The hostess, who lived alone—and was quite beautiful—assured him that if he returned the following day, she would have it there for him. He could not understand why he could not have the coat that moment—and why she was so confident it would be there for him the next day.*
*In one of the great miscalculations of his youth, he sent a friend by to get it for him.*

**A play he had written closed quickly after an out-of-town tryout. Never before had women been more drawn to him. This confirmed his feeling that there existed a small band of women who found failure irresistible.**

He was thrown off stride when a woman he had been pursuing asked him, on their first date, to spank her before they went out to dinner.
He complied, but only halfheartedly. He felt he could have done a much better job of it if they had been a bit further along in their affair. Or at the very least if she'd waited until they had eaten.

He was intrigued by the phenomenon of the *jolie laide* and had met several such women, each of whom was spectacularly ugly. He understood the grotesque appeal of such women, but in the end he decided it was a taste he had no wish to cultivate.

**The sight of a woman dressing was every bit as exciting to him as that of a woman undressing.**

*In Paris, he had slept with a bubble-gum-chewing teenage prostitute while her mother looked on. But he was sick and lonely and miserable at the time and in no mood or position to question the propriety of the encounter.*

He was traveling to Manhattan for emergency dental work when a beautiful young woman boarded the bus and took a seat beside him. He had met her briefly once before and thought of little else in the months that followed. In the course of the trip she made it known to him that, although she was leaving for Europe the following day, she was available to go to bed with him that afternoon. After an agonizing internal debate, he decided to keep his dental appointment. But he never forgave the dentist for allowing his teeth to deteriorate.

**A nondescript woman at a book-signing party instantly captured his attention by mentioning casually that she was an exhibitionist.**

*A friend had taken up with an exquisite stage actress who made his life miserable—drinking to excess, physically assaulting him, torturing him with her infidelities. She turned out to be psychotic and had, eventually, to be put in an institution. Still, he envied the friend for having been with her at all.*

A woman he met at an art gallery in Southampton confessed
that she had always longed to be taken to the beach by
a stranger and made love to—in silence—at the water's edge.
He felt it was an appealing scenario—but the wrong woman.

*His mistress had gained
weight and begun to
neglect her appearance.
Still, he found that he was
able to become aroused—
and to make love to her—
by conjuring up an early
photo on her Washington
State driver's license.*

**He said it often as a joke:
"My fear is that I'll decide
to come out of the closet,
and no one will care."
But, as with all jokes . . .**

**When asked by women
to state his occupation,
he had great success
saying he was a retired
manhunter.**

*Though his politics were,*
*for the most part, liberal—and*
*humanistic—he found*
*right-wing conservative women*
*unbearably attractive.*
*Was it the appeal of the opposite?*
*The slave longing for the lash?*
*Or had his politics become less*
*liberal and humanistic?*

**He postponed a divorce proceeding for six months, because of the magnificent apartment they shared, and its proximity to his favorite delicatessen.**

Remarks that would have been considered gross had they not come from the lips of a beautiful woman:

- *You sure do know how to suck titty.*
- *Butt-fucking? Hey, if you can get past my hems, go for it.*
- *He thought he was some preppy big shot—so I blew him to put him in his place.*

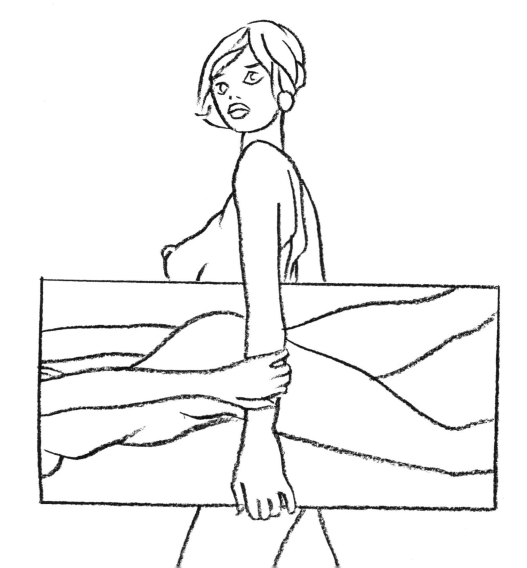

*Her (2)*

She remembered seeing him only once—having drinks with
him, spending the night in his room, and leaving quickly
in the morning. When they met by chance ten years later he
spoke of dinners they had enjoyed, walks in the rain,
all-night carousing, and a magical trip to Cannes.
"You had a tremendous crush on me," he recalled.
She considered correcting him, but decided that doing so
would take longer than the affair itself.

**The most shameful
secret of her life was
that she had gone to
bed with a man after
accepting his (spurious)
claim that he was a
Stroke.**

*She generally gambled in
casinos when she was between
lovers. The hours spent at
the roulette table were relaxing
and relieved her need for sex.
But not entirely.*

*She was pleased when her psychiatrist accepted an invitation to her thirtieth birthday party. Soon after arriving, he drank half a bottle of Absolut vodka, thrust his hand beneath her college classmate's skirt and threw up on an antique rug. When she brought up his behavior at their next session, he denied everything. "You've imagined all this," he insisted, "as part of your resistance to therapy."*

**In a change of style, her lover entered her slowly—exquisitely and almost unbearably so. And she knew, in an instant, that he had been with another woman.**

She'd had her share of affairs, but it crossed her mind—with some disappointment—that none could be regarded as being "steamy."

On the patio of a hotel in Barbados, an elderly New England matron listened to the young man's woeful tale: He had recently learned that his wife had a lover—and had slept with several of his friends. There was also some evidence that she worked part-time as a prostitute. "What you must do," the woman counseled him, "is to arrive home late one night with a spot of lipstick on your collar."

The same woman spoke of her satisfaction with the hotel's masseur. "Of course," she said, "I never allow Toulouse to go under panty."

*During the great Clinton Administration debate, she attempted to refute her friend's position that oral sex was a minor matter, much less serious than sexual intercourse.*
*"Try to imagine a man you adore giving head to another woman."*
*"All right," said the friend, closing her eyes.*
*"And how do you feel about it?"*
*"I'm getting hot."*
*"Oh well," she said, conceding defeat. "There goes that argument."*

**She found herself drawn to a man whose most endearing quality was his ability to listen. Only in time did she realize that he had nothing to say.**

At a charity function, she was introduced to a heavily bejeweled woman with world-weary eyes who might have been a stand-in for Marlene Dietrich in her late years. A baroness, the woman owned a game farm in Tanzania, filmed documentaries on wildlife behavior and had lovers not only in Africa, but also in Hamburg, Kazhakstan and on East Sixtieth Street in Manhattan.

How then was it possible for this woman—with her fascinating background—to be the most boring person she had ever met?

*She was curious about an attractive, accomplished, obviously adoring couple—and wondered what it was that had brought them together. "The first thing I noticed about John," the woman explained, "was that he had a great ass."*

**She had never been able to convince her lovers that her nipples were not particularly sensitive.**

How did her young niece know that six of the boys in her boarding school were no longer virgins?

Each Christmas, for some unfathomable reason, her neighbor in the country—a retired British colonial—came by and presented her with a pair of "Fundees"—underwear that is designed to be worn jointly by a couple. He then invited her to stop by his house and watch lesbian movies.

**She thought back to a party she had given to which she had invited a dozen men, most of whom at one time had been her lover. When only a single fight broke out, she declared the evening a success.**

*She had been told the old poet was mad—but had seen no evidence of it. Then one night, the man turned to her at a dinner party and asked for some insight on why his wife had no interest in cunnilingus, toothlessly miming the act as he spoke. And then cursed her, incomprehensibly, for what he thought was her support for the Kurdish minority in Turkey.*

*When her husband took a lover, she sought out for comfort and*
*advice a friend who was experienced in affairs of the heart.*
*"Do not be overly concerned," the friend assured her. "Such affairs*
*generally peter out after several months."*
*But the friend was wrong. It was the marriage that petered out.*

She was on the brink of starting an affair with a young artist, but
lost her enthusiasm when she was invited to an exhibition of his
work—row upon row of sculpted dishcloths.

**She had never understood
the need for a woman
to fake an orgasm.**

*She could not resist
taking an interest in a
young man who had
been described
as being "hung like a
banana tree."*

*She noticed that whenever she concluded an affair, her closest friend would take up with the (rejected) lover. This amused her. But when the friend found a lover on her own, she became furious.*

**"Can one have sexual relations without actually having sex?" This was the question put to her by a magazine interviewer. "Absolutely not," she answered quickly, and then realized she had become aroused by the voice of the interviewer.**

At college, she wondered about a boy who walked about the campus with a perpetually smug and self-satisfied grin. Years later, she was told by a classmate that the boy had the capability of sucking his own penis.

**An affair was one thing—but she bridled at the thought of having an "extramarital dalliance."**

She'd had a crush on a young novelist for quite some time and finally succeeded in luring him into bed.

But she could not forgive him for folding his pants neatly and placing them on a hanger before he embraced her.

*She was unsure of her abilities as a lover. But she felt that—as in tennis—the more balls you hit, the more your game will improve.*

A young man failed to impress her with the following statement:

"When I go to bed each night, I like nothing more than to curl up with a good work by Heidegger."

**An Italian lover had contrived somehow to suck on both of her nipples simultaneously—which she found fascinating—though not necessarily arousing.**

Only once had she won substantially at blackjack. It was early
evening. She sat alone in a San Juan casino, playing three hands to
amuse herself. She could tell the dealer admired her;
in the most subtle manner, he indicated when it was wise for her
to draw, when it was not. In a brief period of time she won
a great deal of money. But when her lover appeared, the dealer's
face fell, and she felt that she had betrayed him.
Not, of course, to the extent of returning the money.


*She thought back on it as the most agreeable of times. She knew*
*three men, each one accomplished and engaging in a different way.*
*She was a friend to each of them, and on occasion a lover.*
*When she alluded to the arrangement on National Public Radio,*
*the interviewer said her behavior was unconscionable and*
*recommended that she change it immediately.*
*This altered her feelings about National Public Radio.*

HER ( 2 )

At the tip of Miami's
South Beach, which had
become a magnet for models,
she saw an attractive,
well-dressed man of about
sixty, sitting on a
bench and weeping.
"Are you all right?" she asked.
"Yes," he said, through tears.
"Then why are you crying?"
"Because the women are so
beautiful," he said. "And
I can't have them."

**As a young man, he had avoided
an attractive girl at college
because she had the reputation
of being "sexually active."
This was now incomprehensible
to him.**

*He was enamored of a lovely
young television writer and had
the good fortune to meet her
at a cocktail party. He told her
how much he admired her.
"If I were twenty years younger,
I would pursue you relentlessly."
"Why don't you pursue me now,"
she suggested, "only less relentlessly."*

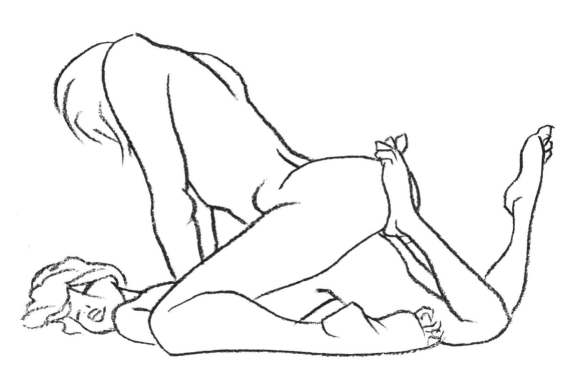

*Twilight*

After a lifetime of what he thought of as a carnal preoccupation with the opposite sex, he came to the surprising conclusion that he enjoyed women because they were more fun than men.

**With the help of Viagra, he returned to sexual form, so to speak, at age seventy. Oddly enough, he had mixed feelings about this sudden renewal.**

Remarks that had been made to him—over the course of a lifetime—that continued to burn in his brain:

- *If you need someone to sleep with you, call me, any hour of the day or night.*
- *Of course I'd like to fuck. What else is there to do?*
- *You poor darling, you haven't had your morning blow job.*

*On balance, pornographic*
*films had had a*
*negative effect on his life.*
*It was not so much*
*the content of them but the*
*chair in which he sat—*
*and his position*
*while he watched—that*
*had caused permanent*
*disability to his back.*

He told a woman he was
no longer able to have sex—
which only increased
her interest in him. This
made him wonder if
impotence did not make
the heart grow fonder.

**He had never known**
**a woman of any age to**
**resent being addressed as**
**"young lady."**

In a novel by Anita Brookner, a sixty-five-year-old man stands naked before a mirror, staring at the reflection of his "irrelevant penis."

No two words in contemporary literature disturbed him more. "Broke-dick"—as the description of a character in Thomas Harris' novel *The Silence of the Lambs*—ran a close second.

**She continued a comfortable but unfulfilling affair, for fear she would die alone—until she realized that she would have to do so in any case.**

*When he turned fifty-six, he became envious of a character in Dostoyevsky's* The Idiot *who was the same age and said to be "in full sap."*

On a summer night in Nantucket, his seventy-year-old
host at a cocktail party, a man he knew only slightly,
said he had some news to share.

"Why don't you join me in my study where we
can speak privately?"

When they were alone, the host said that he had met
and fallen in love with another woman and planned
to leave his wife.

"I have told Betty that I can no longer have sex,"
he whispered.

But then he raised his fist, and in what sounded like a
triumphant battle cry shouted out: "BUT I CAN!"

*He was old and frail and fearful that his young mistress would abandon him. As a final indignity, she forced him to watch repeat episodes of* Touched by an Angel.

A beautiful prostitute had once told him that, after spending three years in the business, she planned to purchase a kennel and raise beagles in the south of Sweden. From time to time, he wondered if she had been able to pull this off.

**When he first tried Viagra, it took effect a day too late—when he was shopping in a hardware store.**

She felt confident that when she reached her advanced years, sex would no longer dominate her thoughts. But she was wrong. Sex, as it always had, created a need for more sex.

*"When you are depressed,"*
*a therapist had told him, "think*
*back to when you last were*
*happy—and try to repeat the*
*circumstances."*
*Since his previous blissful*
*moments had come about when*
*he was rich, famous, had a*
*desirable girlfriend and*
*was twenty-five years younger—*
*the advice was not useful.*

**As he grew older, he begin to cultivate women not as lovers but as friends. In actuality, he had no choice.**

One of the more pleasurable experiences of his life came about when he joined two attractive young women in conversation at a bar in Los Angeles. He was told— after drinks—that they had both fantasized about going to bed with an older man. All three returned to his hotel suite for a magical and exquisite night of sex. Though he did not see the women again, he kept returning to the bar, for a period of twenty years, hoping for a comparable experience, which never took place.

**In his lifetime, there had been women who had spurned him, others who found him appealing—but only one had described him as being "lusty."**

**Watching a panel of women discuss porn was more erotic to him than the porn they were discussing.**

*He had once told a psychiatrist that a woman he was dating kept a full complement of motorized sex toys at her bedside. The psychiatrist jumped to his feet and shouted: "That's the one!"*

He sensed a tectonic change in the culture when he read this on-line ad: "Wanted, room to rent in nice apartment. Not gay, but will deliver blow jobs if required."

And a friend got great results in the personals with the following ad: "Enormously wealthy man with six months to live seeks attractive companion."

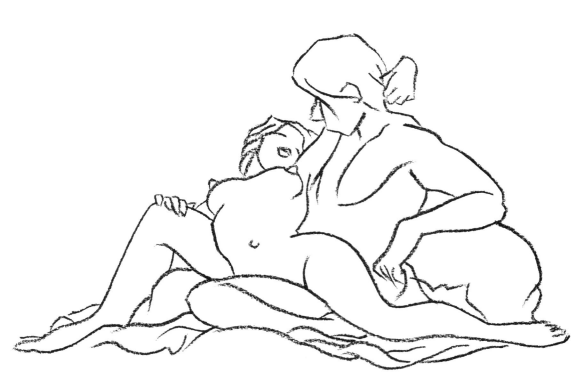

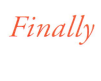

*Finally*

*Though she lived in the moment*
*And speculated little about the future*
*It crossed her mind*
*That there would come a night*
*Or day*
*When she would make love*
*For the last time.*
*Would she be aware*
*That this was happening?*
*Would there be something unique*
*about the experience?*
*apart from the finality of it . . .*

*And where would all this take place?*
*In her apartment in Manhattan?*
*Or in Venice—as she supposed?*
*Her own little death*
*in that sad and fabled city.*

*If she could know all this in advance*
*How would she arrange the encounter?*
*What, for example, would she ask for in bed?*
*Or offer?*
*Something she'd never done?*

*Some interest that had to be addressed?*
*Or would she be silent,*
*allowing the adventure simply to unfold?*

*Would she, incidentally,*
*be "restricted" to one orgasm?*
*And would there be music?*
*Church music?*
*Certainly not Rodgers and Hart,*
*certainly not on this occasion.*
*Would her situation*
*Resemble that of a condemned individual*
*Ordering a last meal?*

*And the big question, of course:*
*Who would be her lover?*

Each day he sat in the piazza

Sipped a Negroni

And waited for the Contessa to arrive.

Years before, he had betrayed her

Stolen her youth

Or so she claimed.

Now he'd come to beg her forgiveness

No longer seeking her beauty,

her fragrance,

her great spirit.

Needing only to hold her hand

so that he would not have to die alone.

Months passed.
The Contessa failed to come
And death drew near.
But God was merciful
And infinitely wise.
On the way to the piazza one day
As he smoked a rich cigar
He was struck by a Fiat
And killed instantly—
Obliterated.
So that when the Contessa finally arrived
There was no hand for her to hold.

**Bruce Jay Friedman** has published eight novels, four story collections, and three works of nonfiction, as well as writing a half dozen plays and receiving several screenwriting credits, including *Stir Crazy*, *Doctor Detroit*, and *Splash*, which won him an Academy Award nomination for Best Original Screenplay. His work *The Lonely Guy's Book of Life* provided the basis for Steve Martin's film *The Lonely Guy*.

**André Barbe**, a Parisian artist, has been widely published in French and international periodicals. He has published sixteen books, often animates for film and television, and has mounted one-man exhibitions at leading museums throughout Europe.